Table Of Contents

Flex and Flow: Yoga and Flexibility Training for Adults

Flex and Flow: Yoga and Flexibility Training for Adults

Chapter 1: Introduction to Yoga and Flexibility Training

The Benefits of Yoga and Flexibility Training for Adults

In our fast-paced and stressful modern lives, finding ways to maintain a healthy body and mind is crucial. Yoga and flexibility training offer adults a multitude of benefits that go beyond just physical fitness. In this subchapter, we will explore the numerous advantages of incorporating these practices into your daily routine.

First and foremost, yoga and flexibility training promote physical well-being. By engaging in regular practice, adults can improve their overall flexibility, balance, and strength. As we age, our bodies naturally become less supple, leading to a higher risk of injuries and decreased mobility. However, with consistent yoga and flexibility training, adults can counteract these effects, maintaining their range of motion and reducing the likelihood of muscle strain.

Flex and Flow: Yoga and Flexibility Training for Adults

Moreover, these practices have a profound impact on mental health. Yoga and flexibility training are known for their stress-relieving properties. Through the combination of deep breathing, meditation, and mindful movement, adults can experience a significant reduction in anxiety and an increase in overall well-being. The mind-body connection cultivated in these practices allows individuals to focus on the present moment and let go of negative thoughts, promoting a sense of calm and inner peace.

Additionally, yoga and flexibility training can complement other forms of exercise. For those interested in Pilates and core strengthening, incorporating yoga and flexibility training into your routine can enhance overall performance and prevent injuries. The increased flexibility acquired through these practices allows for a greater range of motion, improving the effectiveness of core exercises and minimizing strain on the muscles.

Furthermore, yoga and flexibility training foster mindfulness in fitness. By bringing awareness to each movement and breath, adults can develop a deeper understanding of their bodies and their limits. This mindfulness carries over into other areas of life, allowing individuals to approach challenges with a calm and focused mindset.

In conclusion, the benefits of yoga and flexibility training for adults are vast. From physical well-being to mental health and mindfulness, these practices offer a holistic approach to fitness. By incorporating yoga and flexibility training into your daily routine, you can experience improved flexibility, reduced stress levels, and enhanced overall wellness. So, take a step towards a healthier and more balanced life by embracing the transformative power of yoga and flexibility training.

Understanding the Mind-Body Connection in Fitness

In the world of fitness, it is not uncommon to focus solely on physical strength and endurance. However, there is a powerful connection between the mind and the body that is often overlooked. This subchapter aims to shed light on this crucial connection and its significance in achieving overall well-being through yoga and flexibility training.

Yoga and flexibility training have long been celebrated for their ability to improve physical strength, flexibility, and balance. But what sets them apart from other forms of exercise is their emphasis on the mind-body connection. Practitioners of yoga and flexibility training understand that the body is not a separate entity from the mind but rather an integral part of it.

Flex and Flow: Yoga and Flexibility Training for Adults

When we engage in yoga poses or flexibility exercises, we are required to be present and fully aware of our bodies. This mindfulness allows us to notice any tension, discomfort, or limitations within our physical bodies. By acknowledging these sensations, we can begin to understand the underlying emotional and psychological factors that may be contributing to them.

Stress, anxiety, and negative emotions can manifest themselves in physical symptoms like tight muscles or shallow breathing. Through yoga and flexibility training, we learn to cultivate self-awareness and release these emotions, ultimately improving our physical well-being. By consciously connecting our minds to our bodies, we can identify areas of tension and work towards releasing them, promoting relaxation and a sense of calm.

Moreover, the mind-body connection in fitness extends beyond the physical realm. It also plays a vital role in enhancing our overall mental health and well-being. Yoga and flexibility training offer a safe space for self-reflection and introspection. By incorporating mindfulness techniques such as deep breathing and meditation into our practice, we learn to quiet the mind, reduce stress, and cultivate a positive mental state.

In a world that often demands constant productivity and multitasking, the mind-body connection becomes even more critical. By engaging in yoga and flexibility training, we give ourselves permission to slow down, tune into our bodies, and reconnect with ourselves on a deeper level. This connection allows us to not only improve our physical fitness but also enhance our mental clarity, emotional resilience, and overall quality of life.

In conclusion, understanding and nurturing the mind-body connection is essential in achieving holistic well-being through yoga and flexibility training. By embracing mindfulness and self-awareness, we can unlock the true potential of our bodies and minds, leading to improved physical fitness, mental health, and a greater sense of balance in our lives.

Chapter 2: Getting Started with Yoga

The Basics of Yoga

Yoga is an ancient practice that has been embraced by millions of individuals around the world for its numerous physical, mental, and spiritual benefits. In this subchapter, we will delve into the basics of yoga, providing you with a solid foundation to begin or enhance your yoga journey.

Yoga and flexibility training go hand in hand, making it an ideal choice for those seeking to improve their flexibility. Flexibility is not only crucial for preventing injuries during physical activities but also for maintaining joint health and overall mobility. Yoga poses, or asanas, gently stretch and lengthen the muscles, improving flexibility over time. Whether you're a beginner or have some experience, we will guide you through a series of beginner-friendly asanas, ensuring that you progress at your own pace.

Pilates and core strengthening enthusiasts will also find value in yoga. While Pilates primarily focuses on strengthening the core muscles, yoga takes a holistic approach by targeting the entire body. Through a combination of standing, seated, and supine poses, yoga engages the core while also working the muscles in the arms, legs, and back. By incorporating yoga into your routine, you will not only strengthen your core but also develop a strong, balanced physique.

Beyond physical fitness, yoga emphasizes the mind-body connection and mindfulness in fitness. In today's fast-paced world, it is essential to cultivate a sense of mindfulness and be present in the moment. Yoga encourages this by incorporating breath control and meditation into the practice. As you flow through the asanas, you will learn to synchronize your breath with your movements, promoting a sense of calm and inner peace. Additionally, yoga teaches you to listen to your body and honor its limitations, fostering a deeper understanding of yourself and your capabilities.

No matter your age or fitness level, yoga is a practice that can be tailored to suit your individual needs. It offers a gentle yet effective approach to improving flexibility, strengthening the core, and cultivating mindfulness. So, whether you're a seasoned yogi or new to the mat, the basics of yoga will provide you with a solid foundation from which you can build a strong and fulfilling yoga practice.

Yoga Poses for Beginners

In this subchapter, we will explore a range of yoga poses specifically designed for beginners. Whether you are new to yoga or looking to refine your practice, these poses will help you build strength, flexibility, and balance while fostering a mind-body connection.

1. Mountain Pose (Tadasana): Start by standing tall with your feet hip-width apart. Ground yourself and engage your core. This pose improves posture and increases body awareness.

2. Downward-Facing Dog (Adho Mukha Svanasana): From a tabletop position, lift your hips up and back, forming an inverted V-shape with your body. This pose stretches the hamstrings, calves, and shoulders while strengthening the arms and legs.

3. Warrior I (Virabhadrasana I): Step one foot forward into a lunge position, with your back foot at a slight angle. Raise your arms overhead and gaze forward. Warrior I builds strength in the legs and improves balance.

4. Tree Pose (Vrksasana): Stand tall and shift your weight onto one leg. Place the sole of your opposite foot on your inner thigh or calf, avoiding the knee joint. Bring your hands to prayer position in front of your heart. Tree Pose enhances balance and concentration.

5. Child's Pose (Balasana): Start by kneeling on the floor and gently lower your torso to rest between your thighs. Extend your arms forward or alongside your body. This pose promotes relaxation and relieves stress.

6. Bridge Pose (Setu Bandhasana): Lie on your back with knees bent and feet flat on the floor. Lift your hips off the ground, pressing through your feet and engaging your glutes. Bridge Pose strengthens the back and opens the chest.

These are just a few examples of beginner-friendly yoga poses that can be incorporated into your practice. Remember to listen to your body and modify as needed. As you progress, you can gradually challenge yourself with more advanced poses.

By practicing these yoga poses regularly, you will experience improved flexibility, increased strength, and enhanced mind-body connection. Whether you aim to complement your existing fitness routine, find relaxation, or explore mindfulness, yoga offers a multitude of benefits for adults of all fitness levels.

In the next subchapter, we will delve into the world of Pilates and core strengthening exercises that can be combined with your yoga practice to further enhance your overall fitness journey.

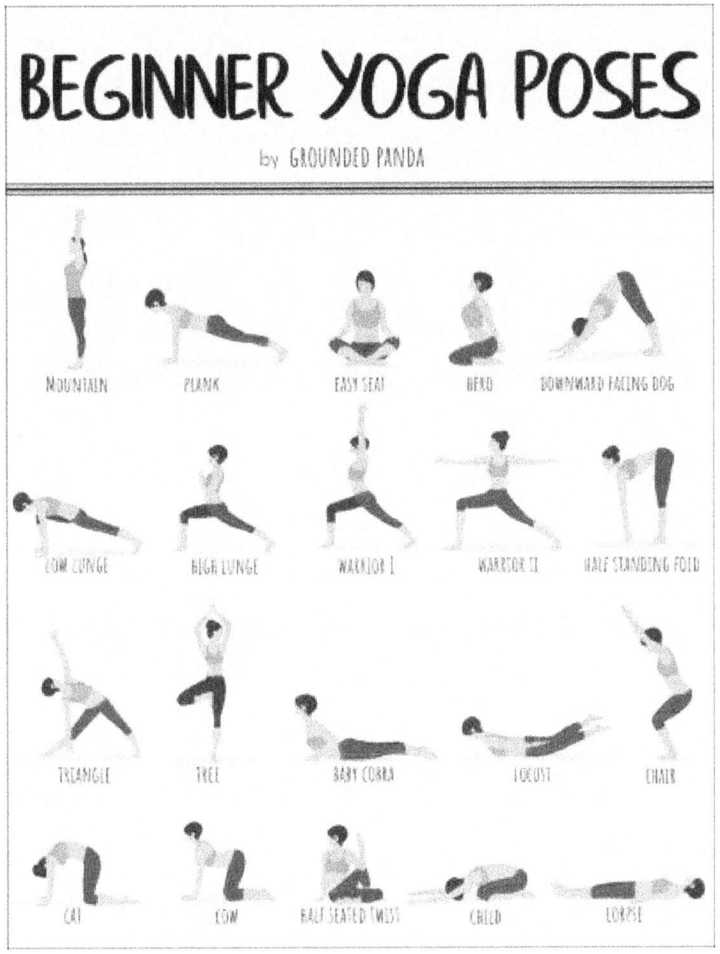

Breathing Techniques in Yoga

In the world of yoga, breath is considered the life force that connects the body, mind, and spirit. The art of controlling the breath is an essential aspect of yoga practice, and mastering different breathing techniques can greatly enhance your yoga experience. This subchapter will delve into the various breathing techniques used in yoga, their benefits, and how to incorporate them into your practice.

One of the fundamental breathing techniques in yoga is called "Ujjayi breath," also known as the victorious breath. Ujjayi breath involves inhaling and exhaling deeply through the nose while slightly constricting the back of the throat. This technique creates a gentle oceanic sound, which helps to focus the mind and deepen the breath. Ujjayi breath is often used during asana practice (yoga postures) to cultivate strength, stability, and concentration.

Another popular breathing technique is "Kapalabhati," the skull-shining breath. Kapalabhati involves forceful exhalations through the nose, while the inhalation is passive. This technique helps to cleanse the respiratory system and energize the body. Kapalabhati is often practiced as a warm-up or as part of a breathing exercise sequence.

Flex and Flow: Yoga and Flexibility Training for Adults

"Anulom Vilom," or alternate nostril breathing, is a technique that helps balance the flow of energy through the body. By using the thumb and ring finger to alternate closing the nostrils, you inhale through one nostril and exhale through the other. This technique promotes relaxation, reduces stress, and enhances mental clarity.

Box breathing, also known as square breathing, is a simple yet powerful technique that involves inhaling, holding the breath, exhaling, and holding again, all for an equal count of seconds. This technique helps to regulate the breath, calm the nervous system, and promote a sense of grounding and focus.

Incorporating these breathing techniques into your yoga practice can deepen your mind-body connection, increase your flexibility, and enhance your overall well-being. By consciously focusing on the breath, you can bring awareness to each movement and transition, allowing you to experience yoga as a moving meditation. Whether you are new to yoga or a seasoned practitioner, exploring and mastering these breathing techniques will undoubtedly enrich your yoga journey.

Remember, yoga is not just about physical flexibility. It is a holistic practice that encompasses the mind, body, and spirit. By embracing the power of breath, you can tap into a deeper level of self-awareness and mindfulness within your yoga and flexibility training.

Yoga Props and Equipment

In the world of yoga and flexibility training, there are a variety of props and equipment that can enhance your practice and take it to the next level. These tools not only provide support and stability but also help in deepening your stretches, improving alignment, and increasing overall strength and flexibility. Whether you are a beginner or an experienced yogi, incorporating yoga props and equipment into your routine can offer numerous benefits.

One of the most commonly used props in yoga is the yoga mat. A good quality mat provides cushioning and grip, ensuring that you have a stable and comfortable surface to perform your poses. It also helps in preventing injuries by providing traction and reducing the risk of slipping.

Blocks and straps are two other essential props that can assist in achieving proper alignment and increasing flexibility. Blocks can be used to support the body in various poses, allowing you to maintain balance and stability. Straps, on the other hand, can be used to deepen stretches and improve flexibility by providing a gentle pull or assistance.

Bolsters and blankets are great props for relaxation and restorative yoga practices. They offer support to the body, allowing you to fully relax into poses and release tension. Bolsters can be used under the knees, back, or neck to promote comfort and relaxation, while blankets can be folded or rolled up to provide additional support or cushioning.

For those looking to challenge their practice and build strength, resistance bands and yoga wheels are excellent options. Resistance bands can be used to add resistance to your yoga poses, making them more intense and engaging different muscle groups. Yoga wheels, on the other hand, can help with deep backbends, core strengthening, and balance.

Incorporating props and equipment into your yoga practice not only enhances your physical capabilities but also deepens your mind-body connection. By using props, you can focus more on your breath, alignment, and the sensations in your body, fostering mindfulness and presence.

Whether you are a yoga enthusiast, a Pilates practitioner, or someone looking to strengthen their core and improve flexibility, investing in a few key yoga props and equipment can greatly enhance your practice. From mats and blocks to resistance bands and bolsters, these tools can help you achieve your fitness and wellness goals while ensuring safety and support. So, don't hesitate to explore the wide range of yoga props available and find the ones that best suit your needs and preferences.

Chapter 3: Developing Flexibility through Yoga

The Science of Flexibility Training

Flexibility training is a crucial component of any fitness routine, whether you are a dedicated yogi, a Pilates enthusiast, or simply someone looking to improve your overall fitness level. Understanding the science behind flexibility training can help you maximize your results and prevent injuries. In this subchapter, we will delve into the science of flexibility training and its benefits for adults in the niches of yoga and flexibility training, Pilates and core strengthening, and the mind-body connection and mindfulness in fitness.

Flexibility refers to the range of motion in your joints and muscles. It is influenced by various factors, including genetics, age, and physical activity level. However, flexibility can be improved through regular training. Flexibility training involves stretching exercises that target specific muscles and joints, helping to increase their range of motion.

Flex and Flow: Yoga and Flexibility Training for Adults

Research has shown that regular flexibility training offers numerous benefits for adults. It can improve posture, balance, and coordination, reducing the risk of falls and injuries. It also enhances athletic performance by improving muscle function and efficiency. Flexibility training can alleviate muscle soreness and tension, increase blood flow to the muscles, and promote relaxation.

For those engaged in yoga and flexibility training, understanding the science behind stretching is essential. The two main types of stretching are static and dynamic. Static stretching involves holding a stretch for an extended period, while dynamic stretching involves moving your joints and muscles through a full range of motion. Both have their benefits and should be incorporated into your practice.

In the niche of Pilates and core strengthening, flexibility training plays a significant role. Pilates exercises focus on strengthening the core muscles while also promoting flexibility and mobility. By incorporating flexibility training into your Pilates routine, you can improve your overall stability, posture, and body alignment.

Moreover, flexibility training is closely linked to the mind-body connection and mindfulness in fitness. When you engage in flexibility exercises, you become more aware of your body and its movement. This mindfulness can help reduce stress, improve focus, and enhance the mind-body connection. By combining flexibility training with techniques like deep breathing and meditation, you can create a holistic fitness practice that benefits both your physical and mental well-being.

In conclusion, the science of flexibility training is a valuable aspect of any fitness routine, particularly in the niches of yoga and flexibility training, Pilates and core strengthening, and the mind-body connection and mindfulness in fitness. By understanding the principles behind flexibility training, you can optimize your workouts, prevent injuries, and achieve a greater level of flexibility, strength, and overall well-being.

Stretching Techniques for Improved Flexibility

Flexibility is a key component of overall fitness and plays a crucial role in preventing injuries, improving posture, and enhancing athletic performance. In this subchapter, we will explore various stretching techniques that can help adults improve their flexibility and achieve a greater range of motion. Whether you are a yoga enthusiast, a Pilates practitioner, or simply someone interested in improving your mind-body connection, these techniques will be beneficial for you.

1. Dynamic Stretching: This type of stretching involves moving parts of your body through a full range of motion. Dynamic stretching is ideal for warming up before a workout or any physical activity. It helps increase blood flow to the muscles, preparing them for the upcoming movements. Examples include arm circles, leg swings, and walking lunges.

2. Static Stretching: This technique involves holding a stretch for a certain period of time, typically around 30 seconds. Static stretches are useful for improving flexibility and increasing muscle length. They are best performed after a workout or physical activity when your muscles are warm. Examples include hamstring stretches, quadriceps stretches, and shoulder stretches.

3. Proprioceptive Neuromuscular Facilitation (PNF): PNF stretching involves a combination of contracting and relaxing muscles to enhance flexibility. It is highly effective in improving range of motion and can be done with a partner or by using a prop like a resistance band. PNF stretching targets specific muscle groups and is often used in rehabilitation settings.

4. Yoga Asanas: Yoga is renowned for its ability to improve flexibility, balance, and strength. Incorporating yoga asanas or poses into your routine can help you achieve a greater range of motion. Poses like downward dog, cobra, and pigeon pose can stretch multiple muscle groups simultaneously, promoting flexibility and mind-body connection.

5. Pilates Stretches: Pilates focuses on core strengthening and stability, but it also offers various stretching exercises to improve flexibility. Moves such as the spine stretch forward, swan dive, and mermaid stretch target specific muscle groups, contributing to overall flexibility and posture improvement.

Remember, consistency is key when it comes to improving flexibility. Aim to stretch at least two to three times per week, gradually increasing the duration and intensity of your stretches. Be mindful of your body's limitations and avoid overstretching, as it may lead to injuries. Listen to your body and respect its boundaries.

Incorporating stretching techniques into your fitness routine will not only enhance your flexibility but also deepen your mind-body connection. Embrace the journey towards greater flexibility and enjoy the benefits it brings to your overall well-being.

Developing a Safe and Effective Flexibility Routine

In the quest for a healthy and balanced lifestyle, it is essential to incorporate flexibility training into your fitness routine. Flexibility not only enhances physical performance but also promotes mental well-being and overall mind-body connection. Whether you are a yoga enthusiast, Pilates practitioner, or simply someone looking to improve your flexibility, developing a safe and effective flexibility routine is crucial for achieving optimal results.

Flex and Flow: Yoga and Flexibility Training for Adults

First and foremost, it is important to prioritize safety when embarking on a flexibility journey. Always warm up before starting any flexibility exercises to prepare your muscles for the demands ahead. Begin with a gentle cardiovascular activity such as brisk walking or light jogging to increase blood flow and raise your body temperature. This will help prevent injuries and ensure that your muscles are adequately prepared for stretching.

When designing your flexibility routine, focus on a variety of stretches that target different muscle groups. Incorporate both static and dynamic stretches to improve range of motion and enhance muscle elasticity. Static stretches involve holding a stretch for a prolonged period, while dynamic stretches involve controlled movements that take the muscles through a full range of motion. By combining both types of stretches, you can effectively improve flexibility while minimizing the risk of muscle strain.

In addition to incorporating different types of stretches, it is crucial to listen to your body and avoid pushing yourself too far. Flexibility gains take time and patience, and forcing yourself into deep stretches can lead to injury. Instead, focus on gradually increasing the intensity and duration of your stretches over time. This gradual approach will allow your muscles and connective tissues to adapt and become more flexible safely.

To further enhance the effectiveness of your flexibility routine, consider incorporating mindfulness techniques. Mind-body connection is an integral part of flexibility training, as it allows you to be fully present in the moment and tune into your body's needs. Practice deep breathing, meditation, or visualization exercises during your flexibility routine to enhance relaxation and promote a deeper stretch.

Remember, flexibility training is a lifelong practice, and consistency is key. Aim to incorporate flexibility exercises into your routine at least three to four times a week to achieve noticeable improvements. As you progress, consider seeking guidance from a qualified instructor or attending classes to ensure proper form and technique.

By developing a safe and effective flexibility routine, you can unlock the full potential of your body, improve your performance in other physical activities, and cultivate a deeper mind-body connection. Embrace the journey, be patient with yourself, and enjoy the transformative benefits that flexibility training brings to your life.

Chapter 4: Advanced Yoga Poses for Flexibility

Challenging Yoga Poses for Experienced Practitioners

In the world of yoga and flexibility training, there comes a time when practitioners seek a new level of challenge to push their bodies and minds further. This subchapter explores some of the most demanding yoga poses that are specifically designed for experienced practitioners. These poses require a high level of strength, flexibility, and concentration, making them perfect for those who have mastered the basics of yoga and are ready to take their practice to new heights.

One challenging pose is the Handstand (Adho Mukha Vrksasana). This pose requires a strong core, stable shoulders, and exceptional balance. By inverting the body, handstands provide numerous benefits such as improved circulation, increased upper body strength, and enhanced focus. However, it is important for experienced practitioners to approach this pose with caution and under the guidance of a qualified instructor.

The Firefly Pose (Tittibhasana) is another challenging pose that demands both strength and flexibility. This arm balance requires practitioners to balance their body weight on their hands while extending their legs straight out in front of them. Firefly Pose strengthens the arms, wrists, and core muscles, while also stretching the hamstrings and inner thighs.

For those seeking a deep stretch and a challenge for the hips, the Compass Pose (Parivrtta Surya Yantrasana) is an excellent choice. This pose requires a combination of hip flexibility, core strength, and balance. Compass Pose helps to open up the hips, stretch the hamstrings, and improve overall balance and stability.

In addition to physical challenges, experienced practitioners often seek poses that deepen their mindfulness and mind-body connection. The Crow Pose (Bakasana) is a powerful arm balance that not only strengthens the arms and wrists but also requires intense focus and concentration. This pose helps practitioners develop a strong mind-body connection by teaching them to trust their physical abilities and overcome fear.

As with any advanced poses, it is crucial for experienced practitioners to approach them mindfully and with proper guidance. It is recommended to practice under the supervision of a knowledgeable instructor who can provide adjustments and support to prevent injuries.

In conclusion, these challenging yoga poses are specifically designed for experienced practitioners who are seeking to take their practice to new heights. They offer physical, mental, and spiritual benefits, pushing the boundaries of strength, flexibility, and mindfulness. Remember to approach these poses with patience, respect your body's limits, and always prioritize safety in your practice.

Deepening Your Flexibility with Advanced Poses

In the journey towards enhancing flexibility and achieving a greater range of motion, advanced poses can serve as a powerful tool. These poses not only challenge your body but also test your mental strength, helping you reach new levels of flexibility and overall well-being. In this subchapter, we will explore how you can deepen your flexibility through advanced poses, allowing you to transcend your current limitations and embrace your full potential.

Advanced poses require a solid foundation in basic yoga and flexibility training. It is essential to have a strong understanding of alignment, proper breathing techniques, and body awareness before attempting these challenging postures. Regular practice of foundational poses prepares your body for the demands of advanced poses and reduces the risk of injury.

Flex and Flow: Yoga and Flexibility Training for Adults

One of the key elements in deepening flexibility through advanced poses is patience. Unlike basic poses, advanced postures cannot be achieved overnight. They require consistent practice, perseverance, and a willingness to step out of your comfort zone. By gradually progressing towards more challenging poses, you can build the strength and flexibility necessary to perform them safely and effectively.

In this subchapter, we will introduce you to a variety of advanced poses that target different areas of the body, including backbends, inversions, and balancing poses. Each pose will be accompanied by detailed instructions, modifications, and alignment cues to ensure proper execution. Additionally, we will provide tips and techniques to gradually work your way into these poses, allowing you to develop the necessary strength and flexibility over time.

Furthermore, we will explore the mind-body connection and mindfulness in the context of advanced poses. Deepening your flexibility goes beyond physical changes; it also involves cultivating a positive mindset and developing mental resilience. Through mindfulness practices such as breathwork and meditation, you can enhance your focus, reduce stress, and improve your overall well-being.

Whether you are a dedicated yogi, a Pilates enthusiast, or someone interested in strengthening their core and improving flexibility, this subchapter will provide you with the tools and knowledge to deepen your flexibility through advanced poses. By embracing the challenges and pushing the boundaries of what you thought was possible, you can unlock a new level of physical and mental freedom. Let us embark on this transformative journey together and discover the true potential of your body and mind.

Precautions and Modifications for Advanced Poses

As you progress in your yoga and flexibility training journey, you may find yourself drawn to challenging and advanced poses. These poses not only require strength and flexibility but also a deep understanding of your body's capabilities. In this subchapter, we will discuss the precautions and modifications you should consider when attempting advanced poses, ensuring that you practice safely and avoid any potential injuries.

First and foremost, it is crucial to listen to your body and respect its limits. Pushing yourself beyond what feels comfortable can lead to strains, sprains, or even more severe injuries. Always warm up properly before attempting any advanced pose and take the time to stretch and prepare the specific muscles involved.

Another important precaution is to have a qualified instructor or spotter present when attempting advanced poses. They can provide guidance, correct your form, and offer modifications tailored to your abilities. Don't hesitate to ask for assistance or feedback; it can make a significant difference in your practice.

When attempting advanced poses, modifications are often necessary to adapt the pose to your body's needs and limitations. For example, if you're working on a challenging arm balance, you can start by using props such as blocks or straps to provide support and stability. Gradually, as your strength and balance improve, you can reduce the assistance from props.

Additionally, always remember to engage your core muscles during advanced poses. Pilates and core strengthening exercises can greatly enhance your stability and control, reducing the risk of injury. Focus on activating your deep abdominal muscles, lower back, and pelvic floor muscles to create a strong and stable foundation for your advanced poses.

Mindfulness plays a crucial role in your practice, particularly when attempting advanced poses. Pay attention to your breath and stay present in the moment, allowing yourself to fully experience the pose without judgment or self-criticism. Be patient with your progress and avoid comparing yourself to others; everyone's journey is unique.

In conclusion, advanced poses can be exhilarating and rewarding, but they require caution and modifications to ensure your safety. Always prioritize listening to your body, seek guidance from qualified instructors, and be mindful of your limitations. By practicing with these precautions in mind, you can continue to deepen your yoga and flexibility training journey while minimizing the risk of injury.

Chapter 5: Pilates and Core Strengthening

Introduction to Pilates and Its Benefits

Pilates is a mind-body exercise system that focuses on core strength, flexibility, and overall body awareness. Developed by Joseph Pilates in the early 20th century, this unique form of exercise has gained popularity among adults seeking to improve their physical fitness, posture, and mental well-being. In this subchapter, we will explore the origins of Pilates, its key principles, and the numerous benefits it offers to individuals of all ages and fitness levels.

Pilates is often described as a fusion of yoga, ballet, and gymnastics, as it incorporates elements from these disciplines to create a comprehensive workout. It emphasizes the importance of proper alignment, controlled movements, and breath control, all of which contribute to a stronger, more balanced body. Unlike traditional weightlifting or cardiovascular exercises, Pilates is a low-impact workout that focuses on quality of movement rather than quantity.

One of the core principles of Pilates is the activation of the body's deep stabilizing muscles, particularly those in the abdomen, lower back, and pelvic floor. By strengthening these muscles, Pilates helps improve overall posture and stability, reducing the risk of injuries and chronic pain. Additionally, Pilates exercises promote better balance, coordination, and flexibility, making it an ideal choice for individuals involved in yoga and flexibility training.

Beyond the physical benefits, Pilates also nurtures the mind-body connection and promotes mindfulness in fitness. Each exercise in Pilates requires concentration, control, and an awareness of one's body in space. By practicing Pilates, individuals can develop a greater sense of body awareness, allowing them to move more efficiently and with more grace in their daily lives.

The benefits of Pilates are numerous and wide-ranging. Regular practice can lead to improved muscle tone, increased flexibility, enhanced athletic performance, and a more centered and calm mind. It can also help alleviate stress and tension, improve posture-related issues, and aid in injury prevention and rehabilitation. Whether you are a seasoned athlete or a beginner looking to start a fitness journey, Pilates offers something for everyone.

In the following chapters, we will delve deeper into the specific Pilates exercises, techniques, and modifications suitable for adults of all fitness levels. By incorporating Pilates into your fitness routine, you will unlock a world of physical and mental benefits that will empower you to live a healthier, more balanced life. So, let's embark on this exciting journey of Flex and Flow, and discover the transformative power of Pilates.

Core Strengthening Exercises in Pilates

Pilates is a highly effective form of exercise that focuses on strengthening the core muscles of the body. Known for its ability to improve flexibility, posture, and overall strength, Pilates has gained immense popularity among adults seeking a well-rounded fitness routine. In this subchapter, we will delve into the world of core strengthening exercises in Pilates, exploring the various techniques and benefits that this practice offers.

At the heart of Pilates lies the concept of the core, which includes the muscles of the abdomen, back, and pelvic floor. These muscles are essential for maintaining stability, balance, and proper alignment in everyday movements. By incorporating specific exercises that target the core, Pilates helps to strengthen these muscles, resulting in improved posture, reduced back pain, and enhanced overall strength.

One such exercise is the "Hundred," where the practitioner lies on their back and lifts their head, neck, and shoulders off the mat while simultaneously pumping their arms up and down. This exercise not only engages the abdominal muscles but also challenges the breath control and coordination, promoting a harmonious connection between the mind and body.

Another widely practiced exercise in Pilates is the "Plank," which involves assuming a push-up position while engaging the core muscles. This exercise not only strengthens the abdominals but also targets the muscles of the arms, shoulders, and legs, making it a full-body workout. Variations of the plank, such as side planks and knee planks, offer additional challenges and benefits.

The beauty of Pilates lies in its emphasis on the mind-body connection and mindfulness in fitness. Each exercise is performed with precision, control, and conscious breathing, allowing practitioners to cultivate a deep sense of awareness and focus. By bringing attention to the present moment and tuning into the body's sensations, Pilates becomes a meditative practice that enhances overall well-being.

Incorporating core strengthening exercises in Pilates into your fitness routine can bring about transformative results. Whether you are a beginner or an experienced practitioner, these exercises offer a multitude of benefits, including improved posture, increased strength, and enhanced mind-body connection. So, let go of any preconceived notions and embark on a journey of self-discovery through Pilates - a practice that nurtures both your body and mind.

Pilates Mat Exercises

Pilates has gained popularity in recent years for its ability to improve core strength, flexibility, and overall body awareness. In this subchapter, we will explore various Pilates mat exercises that can be incorporated into your yoga and flexibility training routine. These exercises not only target the core but also work on different muscle groups, helping to improve strength, balance, and posture.

One of the fundamental Pilates exercises is the Hundred. This exercise engages the deep core muscles while also promoting controlled breathing and stability. By lying on your back with your legs raised and your head and shoulders lifted off the mat, you can challenge your abdominal muscles and increase your overall body strength.

Another beneficial exercise is the Roll Up. This movement focuses on spinal mobility and stretches the hamstrings and lower back. By lying flat on your back and slowly rolling up to a sitting position, you can strengthen your core and improve your flexibility.

Flex and Flow: Yoga and Flexibility Training for Adults

For those looking to target their glutes and thighs, the Bridge exercise is ideal. By lying on your back with your knees bent and feet flat on the mat, you can lift your hips off the ground, engaging your glutes and hamstrings. This exercise not only strengthens the lower body but also helps to stabilize the pelvis and improve posture.

In addition to these exercises, we will explore various variations and modifications that can be tailored to individual needs and fitness levels. Whether you are a beginner or an experienced practitioner, Pilates mat exercises offer a range of options to challenge and strengthen your body.

Furthermore, Pilates emphasizes the mind-body connection and mindfulness in fitness. By focusing on proper alignment, breath control, and concentration, you can cultivate a deeper awareness of your body and its movements. This mindful approach to exercise can help reduce stress, improve mental clarity, and enhance overall well-being.

In conclusion, incorporating Pilates mat exercises into your yoga and flexibility training routine can offer a multitude of benefits. From strengthening your core and improving flexibility to fostering a mind-body connection, these exercises cater to the specific needs of adults seeking a holistic approach to fitness. Whether you are a yoga enthusiast, Pilates practitioner, or simply looking to enhance your overall well-being, these exercises provide an excellent platform for growth and self-improvement.

Pilates Equipment and Apparatus

In the world of fitness and wellness, Pilates has gained immense popularity for its ability to improve core strength, flexibility, and overall body alignment. While mat exercises form the foundation of Pilates, the use of specialized equipment and apparatus takes the practice to a whole new level. In this subchapter, we will explore the various Pilates equipment and apparatus that can enhance your practice and help you achieve optimal results.

One of the most iconic pieces of Pilates equipment is the reformer. This versatile apparatus consists of a sliding carriage, attached to springs of varying tensions, and is used to perform a wide range of exercises. By utilizing the reformer, you can target specific muscle groups and engage your core in a highly controlled and precise manner. The resistance provided by the springs challenges your strength and stability, promoting muscle tone and improving flexibility.

Another popular Pilates apparatus is the Cadillac, also known as the trapeze table. This multifunctional equipment offers a wide variety of exercises that can be tailored to individual needs and abilities. From stretching and strengthening to spinal decompression and inversion, the Cadillac provides a comprehensive full-body workout. Its versatility and adaptability make it a valuable tool for both rehabilitation and advanced Pilates training.

For those seeking a more challenging workout, the Pilates chair, or Wunda chair, offers a unique experience. This compact apparatus consists of a seat with springs and handles, allowing for a wide range of exercises that target the core, legs, and upper body. The chair's design forces you to engage your stabilizing muscles, enhancing balance, coordination, and overall strength.

In addition to these main pieces of equipment, the Pilates repertoire also includes smaller apparatus such as the magic circle, foam roller, and resistance bands. These tools can be incorporated into mat exercises to provide added resistance, assistance, or proprioceptive feedback, intensifying the workout and targeting specific muscle groups.

Whether you are a beginner or a seasoned practitioner, incorporating Pilates equipment and apparatus into your routine can bring new dimensions to your practice. The controlled movements and unique challenges offered by these tools can help you deepen your mind-body connection, improve your flexibility, and strengthen your core. So, step onto the reformer, embrace the Cadillac, and explore the endless possibilities that Pilates equipment can offer on your journey to enhanced well-being and fitness.

Chapter 6: Enhancing the Mind-Body Connection

Mindful Movement and Fitness

In today's fast-paced world, finding balance and tranquility can be a challenge. However, incorporating mindful movement and fitness practices into your daily routine can greatly enhance your overall well-being. This subchapter explores the powerful combination of yoga and flexibility training, Pilates and core strengthening, as well as the mind-body connection and mindfulness in fitness.

Yoga and flexibility training have long been revered for their ability to foster physical and mental harmony. By practicing various yoga asanas (poses) and engaging in regular stretching exercises, adults can improve their flexibility, strength, and balance. Moreover, these practices promote mindfulness, allowing individuals to focus on the present moment and cultivate a sense of inner peace. Whether you are a beginner or an experienced yogi, this section will guide you on your journey towards increased flexibility and serenity.

Pilates and core strengthening exercises are also essential components of a well-rounded fitness routine. By targeting the deep muscles of the abdomen, lower back, and pelvic floor, Pilates helps to develop a strong and stable core. This not only improves posture and prevents injuries but also enhances overall physical performance. In this subchapter, you will learn a variety of Pilates exercises that can be easily incorporated into your fitness regimen, providing you with a solid foundation for mindful movement.

Furthermore, we delve into the mind-body connection and the importance of mindfulness in fitness. Mindfulness refers to the practice of bringing one's attention to the present moment, without judgment. By cultivating mindfulness during physical activity, adults can deepen their connection between the mind and body, allowing for enhanced physical performance and a greater sense of overall well-being. This section provides practical tips and techniques to help you incorporate mindfulness into your workouts, ensuring a holistic approach to fitness.

Flex and Flow: Yoga and Flexibility Training for Adults offers a comprehensive guide to mindful movement and fitness. Whether you are seeking to improve your flexibility, strengthen your core, or develop a deeper mind-body connection, this subchapter has something for everyone. Embrace the power of these practices and unlock your true potential for physical and mental well-being.

Incorporating Mindfulness into Yoga and Flexibility Training

In today's fast-paced and hectic world, it's more important than ever to find moments of peace and tranquility. Many adults turn to yoga and flexibility training to not only improve their physical well-being but also to cultivate a deeper mind-body connection. This subchapter explores the powerful practice of mindfulness and how it can be seamlessly incorporated into your yoga and flexibility training routine.

Mindfulness, simply put, is the act of bringing your attention to the present moment with an open and non-judgmental attitude. By practicing mindfulness during your yoga and flexibility training sessions, you can enhance your overall experience and reap even more benefits from these practices.

One way to incorporate mindfulness into your routine is by focusing on your breath. Paying attention to the inhalation and exhalation as you move through different yoga poses or perform flexibility exercises can help you stay present and grounded. Not only does this deepen your mind-body connection, but it also promotes relaxation and reduces stress.

Another way to practice mindfulness during yoga and flexibility training is by bringing awareness to your body sensations. As you stretch and move, notice how your muscles feel, the sensations of tension and release, and any areas of discomfort or tightness. By tuning in to these physical sensations, you can learn to listen to your body's needs and make adjustments accordingly.

Additionally, incorporating mindfulness into your yoga and flexibility training can help you cultivate a sense of gratitude and appreciation for your body's capabilities. Take a moment to express gratitude for the strength and flexibility you have, and acknowledge the progress you make with each practice. This positive mindset can enhance your overall well-being and motivate you to continue your fitness journey.

Practicing mindfulness in yoga and flexibility training also extends beyond the mat. Incorporate mindful eating habits by savoring each bite and fully engaging your senses. Mindful walking or nature hikes can also be a wonderful way to connect with the present moment and find peace in the beauty of the world around you.

By incorporating mindfulness into your yoga and flexibility training routine, you not only enhance the physical benefits but also cultivate a deeper mind-body connection. This subchapter serves as a guide to help you bring mindfulness into your practice, allowing you to find moments of tranquility and enhance your overall well-being. Embrace the power of mindfulness and witness the transformative effects it can have on your yoga and flexibility training journey.

Mindful Eating and Its Impact on Fitness

In the fast-paced world we live in today, it's easy to find ourselves mindlessly consuming food without paying attention to what and how much we are eating. However, the practice of mindful eating has gained significant popularity in recent years, and for good reason. Mindful eating not only promotes a healthier relationship with food but also has a profound impact on our overall fitness levels.

Mindful eating is all about being present in the moment and fully engaging our senses during meals. It involves paying attention to the taste, texture, and aroma of food, as well as our body's hunger and fullness cues. By practicing mindful eating, we can tap into our body's innate wisdom and make choices that support our fitness goals.

One of the key benefits of mindful eating is that it helps us develop a greater appreciation for the food we eat. Rather than mindlessly devouring our meals, we take the time to savor each bite, which can enhance the overall dining experience. This heightened awareness also enables us to make more conscious choices about the foods we consume. We become more attuned to our body's needs and are better able to select nutritious, whole foods that nourish us from the inside out.

Furthermore, mindful eating helps us cultivate a healthier relationship with our bodies. Instead of viewing food as the enemy or something to be controlled, we learn to see it as a source of nourishment and pleasure. This shift in mindset allows us to enjoy meals without guilt or judgment, which can significantly reduce stress levels and improve overall well-being.

When it comes to fitness, mindful eating can also support our physical goals. By paying attention to our body's hunger and fullness cues, we can avoid overeating and better manage portion sizes. This can be particularly beneficial for those looking to lose weight or maintain a healthy weight. Additionally, mindful eating encourages us to eat more slowly and mindfully, which can aid digestion and prevent discomfort during physical activity.

Incorporating mindful eating into our fitness routine can be a transformative practice. By taking the time to truly listen to our bodies and honor its needs, we can enhance our overall well-being and achieve greater fitness success. So, the next time you sit down for a meal, take a moment to pause, breathe, and savor each bite. Your body and mind will thank you.

Chapter 7: Mindfulness Practices for Stress Reduction

The Role of Mindfulness in Stress Management

In today's fast-paced world, stress has become an inevitable part of our daily lives. Juggling work, family, and personal commitments often leaves us feeling overwhelmed and emotionally drained. Many of us turn to various stress management techniques to find relief, but have you ever considered the powerful role mindfulness can play in managing stress?

Mindfulness is a practice that involves bringing one's attention to the present moment, without judgment. It is about cultivating a state of awareness and acceptance of our thoughts, feelings, and sensations. By focusing on the present, mindfulness allows us to detach from the worries of the past or future, bringing a sense of calm and clarity to our minds.

When it comes to stress management, mindfulness can be a game-changer. Research has shown that practicing mindfulness regularly can reduce the levels of stress hormones in our bodies, such as cortisol. By engaging in mindfulness exercises, we can train our minds to respond to stressors in a more composed and balanced manner.

In the realm of yoga and flexibility training, incorporating mindfulness can enhance the overall experience and benefits of your practice. By being fully present during each pose, you can connect with your body on a deeper level, noticing the sensations and exploring your limits with kindness and compassion. This not only improves flexibility but also promotes a sense of calm and relaxation, allowing you to let go of any tension or stress held within your muscles.

Pilates and core strengthening exercises also benefit from the inclusion of mindfulness. By focusing on your breath and maintaining awareness of your body's movements, you can enhance the mind-body connection and improve your overall performance. Mindfulness in core strengthening exercises helps to stabilize the mind and body, allowing for efficient muscle engagement and reducing the risk of injury.

Incorporating mindfulness into your fitness routine is not just about stress management but also about cultivating self-awareness and self-compassion. By being present in the moment, you can better understand your body's needs and limitations, avoiding unnecessary strain or pushing beyond your limits. This mindful approach fosters a loving and nurturing relationship with your body, promoting overall well-being and self-acceptance.

In conclusion, mindfulness plays a vital role in stress management, and its inclusion in yoga, flexibility training, Pilates, and core strengthening exercises can greatly enhance their benefits. By practicing mindfulness, you can reduce stress levels, promote calmness, and develop a deeper mind-body connection. So, take a moment to breathe, be present, and embrace the transformative power of mindfulness in your fitness journey.

Breathing Techniques for Stress Reduction

In today's fast-paced world, stress has become an unavoidable part of our lives. The demands of work, family, and personal responsibilities can leave us feeling overwhelmed and drained. Thankfully, there are effective techniques to help reduce stress, and one of the most powerful tools at our disposal is our breath.

In this subchapter, we will explore various breathing techniques that can be incorporated into your yoga and flexibility training, Pilates and core strengthening routines, or any other mind-body connection and mindfulness practices you engage in. These techniques will not only help you find calm and relaxation but also enhance your overall well-being.

One of the simplest yet most effective techniques is diaphragmatic breathing. By consciously engaging the diaphragm, the muscle responsible for our breath, we can activate the body's relaxation response. To practice this technique, find a comfortable seated or lying position. Close your eyes and place one hand on your belly and the other on your chest. Take a slow, deep breath in through your nose, allowing your belly to rise as you fill your lungs with air. Exhale slowly through your mouth, feeling your belly fall. Repeat this process several times, focusing on the sensation of your breath as it moves in and out.

Another technique that can be particularly beneficial during moments of intense stress is the 4-7-8 breath. This technique involves inhaling for a count of 4, holding the breath for a count of 7, and exhaling slowly for a count of 8. This pattern helps regulate the nervous system and allows you to release tension and anxiety.

In addition to these techniques, alternate nostril breathing can help balance the body's energy and reduce stress. By using your fingers to close one nostril at a time, you can alternate the flow of breath between the left and right nostrils. This practice can bring a sense of harmony and calmness to your mind and body.

Incorporating these breathing techniques into your daily routine can have a profound impact on your stress levels and overall well-being. Whether you are engaging in yoga, Pilates, or any other mind-body practice, taking the time to focus on your breath will allow you to cultivate a deeper connection with yourself and find inner peace. So, take a moment to pause, breathe, and let go of the stress that no longer serves you. Your body and mind will thank you.

Mindfulness Meditation for Relaxation

In today's fast-paced world, finding moments of relaxation and calm can be a challenge. The constant demands of work, family, and daily responsibilities can leave us feeling stressed and overwhelmed. However, there is a powerful tool that can help us find peace and tranquility amidst the chaos – mindfulness meditation.

Mindfulness meditation is a practice that involves focusing your attention on the present moment, without judgment or attachment. It is about being fully present in the here and now, allowing your thoughts and emotions to come and go without getting caught up in them. By cultivating this state of non-judgmental awareness, you can experience deep relaxation and inner peace.

In the subchapter "Mindfulness Meditation for Relaxation" in our book "Flex and Flow: Yoga and Flexibility Training for Adults," we delve into the benefits and techniques of mindfulness meditation specifically tailored for adults engaged in yoga, flexibility training, Pilates, and core strengthening exercises.

One of the primary benefits of mindfulness meditation is stress reduction. Research has shown that regular practice can lower cortisol levels, the hormone associated with stress, and promote a sense of calm and relaxation. By incorporating mindfulness meditation into your fitness routine, you can enhance the overall effectiveness of your workouts while also reaping the mental and emotional benefits.

Our subchapter provides step-by-step guidance on how to practice mindfulness meditation. We explore various techniques, such as body scan meditation, in which you systematically scan your body, paying attention to any sensations or areas of tension. We also delve into breath awareness meditation, where you focus on your breath as it moves in and out of your body, using it as an anchor to the present moment.

Additionally, we offer tips on integrating mindfulness into your daily life. From mindful eating to mindful movement during yoga or flexibility exercises, we explore how to infuse each moment with awareness and intention.

Whether you are a seasoned yogi or new to the world of fitness, incorporating mindfulness meditation into your routine can bring profound benefits. By cultivating a mind-body connection and practicing mindfulness, you can enhance your overall well-being, increase flexibility, and find a deep sense of relaxation in both your body and mind.

Join us on this transformative journey as we explore the power of mindfulness meditation for relaxation. Discover how this ancient practice can help you find serenity amidst the chaos of modern life and unlock the full potential of your mind and body.

Chapter 8: Designing a Personalized Yoga and Flexibility Training Program

Assessing Your Current Flexibility and Fitness Level

Before embarking on a yoga or flexibility training journey, it is essential to assess your current flexibility and fitness level. This self-evaluation will help you understand where you stand physically and mentally, allowing you to set realistic goals and tailor your practice to your individual needs. In this subchapter, we will explore various methods to assess your flexibility and fitness level, ensuring a safe and effective journey towards improved well-being.

Flex and Flow: Yoga and Flexibility Training for Adults

Flexibility Assessment:

Flexibility is a crucial aspect of yoga and flexibility training. To assess your current flexibility, start by performing a series of basic stretches for different muscle groups. Pay attention to how far you can comfortably stretch without feeling any pain or discomfort. Use a flexibility chart or app to measure your range of motion and track your progress over time. Remember, flexibility differs for each individual, so don't compare yourself to others. Instead, focus on your own improvement and celebrate small victories along the way.

Fitness Assessment:

In addition to flexibility, evaluating your overall fitness level is important. Begin by assessing your cardiovascular endurance, which determines how efficiently your heart and lungs can supply oxygen to your muscles during physical activity. You can do this by performing a timed walk or jog and noting how long it takes for you to feel fatigued. Additionally, assess your muscular strength and endurance by performing exercises like squats, push-ups, or planks and noting the number of repetitions you can comfortably complete. Finally, assess your balance and stability through exercises such as standing on one leg or balancing on a stability ball.

Mind-Body Connection Assessment:

Yoga and flexibility training not only focus on physical aspects but also emphasize the mind-body connection. Take a moment to evaluate your mindfulness and presence during physical activities. Are you able to focus solely on your breath and movements without distractions? Are you able to let go of stress and be fully present in the moment? Assessing your mind-body connection will help you identify areas for improvement and allow you to cultivate a deeper sense of mindfulness throughout your practice.

By assessing your current flexibility and fitness level, you gain a clearer understanding of where you are starting from, enabling you to set realistic goals and design a personalized practice. Remember, progress takes time and consistency. Embrace the journey, celebrate your achievements, and always listen to your body's needs. With dedication and patience, you will witness your flexibility, fitness, and mind-body connection flourishing, leading to a healthier and more balanced life.

Setting Realistic Goals and Tracking Progress

In the journey of yoga and flexibility training, it is crucial to set realistic goals and track your progress to ensure continuous growth and improvement. This subchapter will guide you through the process of setting attainable objectives and provide effective strategies to monitor your advancement.

Setting realistic goals is essential for several reasons. First and foremost, it enables you to stay motivated and focused on your practice. By establishing achievable targets, you create a sense of purpose and direction, which encourages you to push yourself further. Whether your goal is to master a specific yoga pose, increase your flexibility, or improve your core strength, setting realistic benchmarks ensures that you are constantly striving for improvement without feeling overwhelmed.

To set realistic goals, start by assessing your current abilities and limitations. Be honest with yourself about your strengths and weaknesses, as this will help you set achievable targets. It is important to remember that progress varies from person to person, so avoid comparing yourself to others. Instead, focus on your own journey and what you want to achieve.

Once you have identified your goals, it is crucial to track your progress. This not only helps you stay on track but also provides a sense of accomplishment and motivation. One effective way to track progress is by maintaining a journal or using a fitness app. Record your practice sessions, noting the poses you attempted, the duration of your sessions, and any improvements you noticed. This will allow you to look back and see how far you have come, boosting your confidence and determination.

Additionally, tracking progress helps identify areas that need extra attention. If you notice a lack of progress in a specific pose or flexibility exercise, you can adjust your training regimen accordingly. Seek guidance from a qualified instructor or consider incorporating additional exercises or modifications to target those areas specifically.

Remember that progress is not always linear. There may be times when you experience setbacks or plateaus, but do not let this discourage you. Stay committed to your practice, trust the process, and celebrate even the smallest achievements along the way.

By setting realistic goals and tracking your progress, you are empowering yourself to reach new heights in your yoga and flexibility training. Embrace the journey, stay dedicated, and watch as your practice evolves and transforms.

Creating a Balanced Routine

In today's fast-paced world, finding balance in our lives can often feel like a daunting task. With the demands of work, family, and personal commitments, it's easy for self-care to take a backseat. However, finding balance is essential for our overall well-being. In this subchapter, we will explore the importance of creating a balanced routine and how it can positively impact our lives.

Flex and Flow: Yoga and Flexibility Training for Adults

Yoga and flexibility training, Pilates and core strengthening, and the mind-body connection are all integral parts of achieving balance. By incorporating these practices into our daily routines, we can cultivate physical and mental strength, flexibility, and mindfulness.

To begin, let's focus on yoga and flexibility training. These practices not only enhance our physical flexibility but also promote mental relaxation and stress reduction. By dedicating a few minutes each day to stretching and yoga poses, we can release tension from our bodies and minds, allowing for improved focus and clarity. Whether it's a gentle flow or a more vigorous practice, the benefits of yoga and flexibility training can be felt throughout our day.

Next, let's explore Pilates and core strengthening. These exercises are designed to build strength, particularly in our core muscles, improving our overall stability and posture. By incorporating Pilates into our routine, we can strengthen our bodies while also preventing injuries. Additionally, these exercises promote body awareness and control, allowing us to move more efficiently throughout our daily activities.

Flex and Flow: Yoga and Flexibility Training for Adults

Lastly, let's delve into the mind-body connection and mindfulness in fitness. By bringing awareness to our breath, thoughts, and sensations during exercise, we can cultivate a deeper connection between our mind and body. This practice encourages us to be present in the moment, enhancing our overall experience and reducing stress. By incorporating mindfulness techniques such as focused breathing and meditation into our routine, we can improve our mental well-being and find greater balance in our lives.

In conclusion, creating a balanced routine is essential for adults seeking to improve their overall well-being. By incorporating practices such as yoga and flexibility training, Pilates and core strengthening, and mindfulness in fitness, we can cultivate physical and mental strength, flexibility, and mindfulness. These practices not only benefit our physical health but also enhance our ability to navigate the challenges of everyday life with ease and grace. Start incorporating these practices into your routine today and experience the transformative power of balance.

Incorporating Variety and Progression in Training

When it comes to achieving optimal fitness and flexibility, it's essential to incorporate variety and progression into your training routine. Whether you're a dedicated yogi, Pilates enthusiast, or someone looking to enhance their mind-body connection, this subchapter will explore the benefits of diversifying your workouts and gradually increasing the intensity to reach new levels of strength and flexibility.

Variety is the spice of life, and this holds true for your fitness journey as well. By incorporating different types of exercises into your routine, you engage multiple muscle groups, prevent boredom, and challenge your body in new ways. For yoga and flexibility training enthusiasts, this could mean exploring different styles of yoga, such as Hatha, Vinyasa, or Ashtanga, to target different areas of the body and promote overall flexibility.

If you're a fan of Pilates and core strengthening, consider incorporating props like resistance bands, stability balls, or Pilates rings to add variety and intensify your workouts. These props not only provide a fresh challenge but also target specific muscles, helping you build a strong and stable core.

Flex and Flow: Yoga and Flexibility Training for Adults

While variety is important, progression is equally crucial for continued growth and improvement. Gradually increasing the intensity, duration, or complexity of your workouts helps push your limits and ensures you don't plateau in your fitness journey. For example, if you've mastered a particular yoga pose, try advancing to a more challenging variation or holding the pose for a longer duration. This progression allows you to continually challenge your body and reach new levels of flexibility and strength.

Additionally, mind-body connection and mindfulness play a vital role in any fitness routine. As adults, we often lead hectic lives filled with stress and distractions. Incorporating mindfulness techniques, such as deep breathing exercises or meditation, into your training sessions can help you stay present, focused, and in tune with your body. This mindfulness not only enhances your overall workout experience but also promotes relaxation and stress reduction.

In summary, incorporating variety and progression in your training routine is key to achieving optimal results in yoga, flexibility training, Pilates, and core strengthening. By diversifying your workouts, gradually increasing the intensity, and staying mindful throughout, you'll not only challenge your body but also cultivate a deeper mind-body connection. So, embrace the journey, try new exercises, and watch as your strength, flexibility, and overall well-being flourish.

Chapter 9: Overcoming Challenges in Yoga and Flexibility Training

Common Obstacles and How to Overcome Them

In the journey towards achieving flexibility and a strong mind-body connection, there are often obstacles that can hinder progress. However, with the right mindset and strategies, these obstacles can be overcome. In this subchapter, we will explore some common obstacles faced by adults in their yoga and flexibility training, Pilates and core strengthening, as well as maintaining a mind-body connection in their fitness routines. We will also provide practical tips on how to overcome these challenges.

One of the most common obstacles encountered by adults in their yoga and flexibility training is a lack of time. The demands of work, family, and other commitments often leave little room for self-care. To overcome this, it is important to prioritize your well-being and carve out dedicated time for your practice. Even just 15 minutes a day can make a significant difference. Consider waking up a bit earlier or finding pockets of time throughout the day to fit in some stretches or yoga poses.

Another obstacle that adults face is the fear of injury. Many individuals worry that they are not flexible enough or that they might strain a muscle. It is crucial to remember that flexibility is a journey and that progress takes time. Start with gentle stretches and gradually increase the intensity as your body allows. Seek guidance from a qualified instructor who can provide modifications and ensure proper alignment to minimize the risk of injury.

For those engaged in Pilates and core strengthening, a common obstacle is lack of motivation or plateauing. To overcome this, try incorporating variety into your routine. Explore different Pilates exercises or core-strengthening techniques to keep things interesting. Set realistic goals and celebrate small achievements along the way. Surround yourself with a supportive community or find an accountability partner who can help you stay motivated and committed to your practice.

Maintaining a mind-body connection and mindfulness in fitness can also be a challenge for adults. The distractions of daily life often make it difficult to stay present during workouts. To overcome this, incorporate mindfulness exercises into your routine. Before starting your practice, take a few moments to focus on your breath and set an intention for your session. Throughout your workout, bring awareness to the sensations in your body and stay present in the moment. Practicing meditation or incorporating mindful movement exercises, such as tai chi or qigong, can also help cultivate a stronger mind-body connection.

In conclusion, while there may be obstacles on the path to achieving flexibility, core strength, and a mindful fitness routine, they can be overcome with perseverance and the right strategies. By prioritizing self-care, seeking guidance, staying motivated, and cultivating mindfulness, adults can unlock the full potential of their yoga and flexibility training, Pilates and core strengthening, and mind-body connection in their fitness journey. Remember, progress takes time, so be patient with yourself and enjoy the process.

Dealing with Physical Limitations and Injuries

In a world where physical fitness is often associated with intense workouts and high-impact exercises, it is important to remember that our bodies have limitations. Whether it's due to a pre-existing condition, an injury, or simply the natural aging process, we all face physical limitations at some point in our lives. However, these limitations do not have to hinder our journey towards health and wellness. With the right mindset and approach, we can still achieve flexibility, strength, and mindfulness through yoga and other forms of exercise.

Yoga and flexibility training offer a unique and gentle way to work with our bodies, regardless of any physical limitations we may have. By focusing on the breath and practicing mindful movements, we can gradually increase our flexibility and strength without placing unnecessary stress on our bodies. This makes yoga an ideal choice for individuals recovering from injuries or dealing with chronic pain.

For those seeking to strengthen their core and improve posture, Pilates is a fantastic option. Pilates exercises focus on engaging the deep muscles of the abdomen and back, helping to support and stabilize the spine. This can greatly benefit individuals with back pain or those looking to prevent future injuries. By incorporating Pilates into our fitness routine, we can develop a strong and balanced core, leading to improved overall strength and stability.

In addition to physical training, it is equally important to cultivate a mind-body connection and practice mindfulness in our fitness journey. Mindfulness allows us to be fully present in the moment, to listen to our bodies, and to make conscious choices that support our overall well-being. By incorporating mindfulness into our yoga or Pilates practice, we can deepen our understanding of our bodies, develop greater body awareness, and prevent potential injuries.

When dealing with physical limitations and injuries, it is crucial to approach our fitness journey with patience, compassion, and acceptance. It's important to remember that progress may be slower than we anticipate, and that's okay. By listening to our bodies and honoring our limitations, we can still experience the incredible benefits of yoga, Pilates, and mindfulness in our lives.

No matter what physical limitations or injuries we may be facing, it is possible to find joy, strength, and healing through movement and mindfulness. Flex and Flow: Yoga and Flexibility Training for Adults offers a comprehensive guide to help individuals navigate their fitness journey, providing modifications and adaptations for different physical abilities. With the right mindset and the support of these practices, we can overcome our limitations and uncover the true potential of our bodies.

Staying Motivated and Consistent in Your Practice

In your journey towards improved flexibility and overall well-being, it is crucial to maintain motivation and consistency in your practice. This subchapter will provide you with valuable insights and practical tips to help you stay on track and achieve your fitness goals.

Motivation is the driving force that propels us forward, even when faced with challenges or obstacles. To stay motivated, it is essential to set clear and realistic goals. Start by identifying what you want to achieve in your yoga and flexibility training, be it increasing your range of motion, improving your balance, or reducing stress. Write down these goals and revisit them regularly to remind yourself of what you are working towards.

Flex and Flow: Yoga and Flexibility Training for Adults

Another effective technique to stay motivated is to vary your practice. Engaging in a diverse range of exercises and activities, such as yoga, Pilates, and core strengthening, not only keeps your routine fresh and exciting but also prevents boredom and plateaus. Experiment with different styles of yoga or try new flexibility training techniques to challenge yourself and keep your motivation levels high.

Consistency is equally important as motivation. Establishing a regular practice schedule is key to making progress and reaping the benefits of your efforts. Consistency helps to build discipline and ensures that you make time for your practice amidst the demands of daily life. Find a time of day that works best for you and commit to it. Treat your practice as a non-negotiable appointment with yourself, and over time, it will become a natural part of your routine.

To maintain consistency, it is crucial to create a supportive environment. Surround yourself with like-minded individuals who share your passion for yoga, flexibility training, and mindfulness in fitness. Join a yoga class, find an accountability partner, or participate in online communities to connect with others who can inspire and motivate you on your journey.

Lastly, embrace the power of mindfulness. Mind-body connection plays a vital role in enhancing your practice and keeping you focused. Incorporate mindfulness techniques, such as deep breathing and meditation, into your routine. By being fully present during your practice, you will experience greater benefits and find it easier to stay consistent and motivated.

Remember, motivation and consistency are the pillars of progress in yoga and flexibility training. By setting clear goals, varying your practice, establishing a routine, creating a supportive environment, and cultivating mindfulness, you will unlock your full potential and achieve remarkable results. Stay committed, stay motivated, and embrace the transformative power of your practice.

Chapter 10: Taking Your Yoga and Flexibility Training to the Next Level

Exploring Advanced Yoga Styles

In the realm of yoga and flexibility training, there are several advanced yoga styles that can take your practice to new heights. These styles not only challenge your physical strength and flexibility but also deepen your mind-body connection and promote mindfulness in fitness. In this subchapter, we will delve into some of these advanced yoga styles that are perfect for adults seeking a more intense and transformative yoga experience.

One of the most popular advanced yoga styles is Ashtanga yoga. This dynamic and physically demanding practice follows a specific sequence of postures that flow together seamlessly. Ashtanga yoga focuses on synchronized breathing, movement, and internal energy locks, known as bandhas, to create a moving meditation. With regular practice, Ashtanga yoga builds strength, flexibility, and endurance, while also nurturing a sense of discipline and self-awareness.

For those looking to combine yoga with core strengthening, Power yoga is an ideal choice. This vigorous and fast-paced style incorporates traditional yoga postures with dynamic movements and strength-building exercises. Power yoga not only increases physical stamina and tones the muscles but also improves mental clarity and focus. It is an excellent option for individuals who enjoy challenging workouts and want to enhance their overall fitness level.

Another advanced yoga style worth exploring is Kundalini yoga. Known as the "yoga of awareness," Kundalini yoga focuses on awakening the dormant energy within the body. This practice involves a series of dynamic movements, breathwork, chanting, and meditation techniques. Kundalini yoga aims to balance the chakras, increase vitality, and promote spiritual growth. It is particularly beneficial for individuals seeking a deeper connection between mind, body, and spirit.

Furthermore, Yin yoga is a gentle yet profound yoga style that targets the connective tissues, such as ligaments and fascia, through long-held passive postures. This practice helps improve flexibility and joint mobility while also cultivating inner stillness and relaxation. Yin yoga is perfect for individuals who want to balance their more active and dynamic fitness routines with a calming and introspective practice.

Exploring advanced yoga styles can bring new dimensions to your yoga and flexibility training journey. Whether you choose the dynamic flow of Ashtanga or Power yoga, the spiritual awakening of Kundalini yoga, or the deep relaxation of Yin yoga, these advanced styles offer a transformative experience for your mind, body, and soul. Embrace the challenge, nurture your inner self, and witness the incredible growth that advanced yoga styles can bring to your overall well-being.

Power Yoga and Its Benefits

In the realm of yoga and flexibility training, Power Yoga has emerged as a dynamic and invigorating practice that offers numerous benefits for adults seeking to enhance their physical fitness and overall well-being. This subchapter delves into the essence of Power Yoga, exploring its origins, principles, and the myriad advantages it brings to practitioners.

Flex and Flow: Yoga and Flexibility Training for Adults

Power Yoga, also known as Vinyasa or Flow Yoga, is a modern yoga style that combines traditional yoga postures with a dynamic and continuous flow of movement. It emphasizes strength, flexibility, and breath control, making it a perfect choice for adults looking for a challenging and holistic fitness regime. Unlike other yoga styles, Power Yoga is less focused on spiritual aspects and more on physicality, making it accessible to a wide range of individuals.

One of the primary benefits of Power Yoga is its ability to build strength and flexibility simultaneously. Through the consistent practice of Power Yoga, adults can develop lean muscle mass, increase endurance, and improve overall body tone. The sequences of flowing movements, combined with mindful breathing techniques, engage multiple muscle groups, resulting in increased core strength, improved posture, and enhanced balance.

Moreover, Power Yoga offers an excellent cardiovascular workout, making it an excellent choice for those aiming to shed excess weight and improve their overall fitness levels. The continuous movement and dynamic transitions in Power Yoga classes elevate heart rate and stimulate the circulatory system, leading to increased calorie burn and improved cardiovascular health.

Beyond the physical benefits, Power Yoga also promotes mental well-being and mindfulness. The emphasis on conscious breathing and the synchronization of breath with movement helps adults cultivate a deep mind-body connection. Regular practice of Power Yoga can reduce stress, anxiety, and promote mental clarity, allowing individuals to find a sense of calm and serenity amidst the chaos of daily life.

Furthermore, Power Yoga can be a gateway to developing mindfulness in fitness. By encouraging practitioners to stay present in the moment and focus on their breath and body sensations, Power Yoga fosters a heightened awareness of the mind-body connection. This mindfulness can extend beyond the yoga mat and be applied to other aspects of life, leading to improved concentration, self-awareness, and overall emotional well-being.

In conclusion, Power Yoga is a captivating and transformative practice that offers a multitude of benefits to adults seeking to enhance their physical fitness, flexibility, and mental well-being. Through its emphasis on strength, flexibility, mindful breathing, and mindfulness in fitness, Power Yoga has the potential to revolutionize one's fitness journey, helping adult practitioners achieve their health and wellness goals while cultivating a deep sense of balance and harmony in their lives.

Yin Yoga for Deep Tissue Stretching

In the bustling world we live in, where stress and tension seem to be constant companions, finding effective ways to relax and unwind is essential for maintaining a healthy mind and body. One such method that has gained popularity in recent years is Yin Yoga. Known for its slow and gentle approach, Yin Yoga offers a unique opportunity to delve deep into our connective tissues and release tension, promoting flexibility, relaxation, and a sense of overall well-being.

Yin Yoga focuses on stretching and lengthening the deep connective tissues within the body, such as ligaments, tendons, and fascia. Unlike other forms of yoga that primarily target muscles, Yin Yoga aims to access the tissues that are often overlooked in our regular fitness routines. By holding poses for an extended period, typically ranging from one to five minutes, Yin Yoga provides a deep and intense stretch that helps to increase flexibility and improve joint mobility.

This subchapter of "Flex and Flow: Yoga and Flexibility Training for Adults" is dedicated to exploring the benefits and techniques of Yin Yoga for deep tissue stretching. Whether you are a yoga enthusiast, someone looking to enhance your flexibility, or seeking a mindful and relaxing fitness practice, this subchapter will provide you with a comprehensive understanding of Yin Yoga and how it can benefit your mind, body, and spirit.

Throughout this chapter, we will delve into various Yin Yoga poses that specifically target different areas of the body, such as hips, lower back, and shoulders. You will learn how to safely enter and exit these poses, and discover modifications and variations that suit your individual needs and abilities.

Additionally, we will explore the mind-body connection and the role of mindfulness in Yin Yoga. By cultivating a sense of awareness and presence during your practice, you will not only experience physical benefits but also gain a deeper understanding of your own body and its unique needs.

Whether you are new to yoga or a seasoned practitioner, the subchapter "Yin Yoga for Deep Tissue Stretching" will provide you with the tools and knowledge to incorporate Yin Yoga into your fitness routine. Embrace the slow, meditative nature of Yin Yoga, and unlock a world of deep relaxation, increased flexibility, and enhanced mind-body connection.

Chapter 11: Yoga and Flexibility Training for Specific Goals

Yoga for Weight Loss and Toning

In today's fast-paced world, maintaining a healthy weight and toning your body can sometimes feel like an uphill battle. Fad diets and extreme workout routines promise quick results, but often leave you feeling depleted and unsatisfied. Enter yoga – the ancient practice that not only promotes physical strength and flexibility but also nourishes your mind and spirit. In this subchapter, we will explore the powerful benefits of yoga for weight loss and toning, helping you achieve a fit and balanced body.

Yoga offers a holistic approach to weight loss and toning, focusing on both the physical and mental aspects of well-being. Through a combination of asanas (poses), pranayama (breathing techniques), and meditation, yoga helps you shed unwanted pounds while building lean muscle mass. Unlike high-intensity workouts that put stress on your body, yoga provides a gentle yet effective way to burn calories and improve metabolism. Its emphasis on mindful movement and breath control ensures a safe and sustainable weight loss journey.

One of the key benefits of yoga for weight loss is its ability to reduce stress and emotional eating. By incorporating mindfulness and deep breathing, yoga helps you connect with your body and recognize true hunger signals. As you become more aware of your emotions, you can curb impulsive eating habits and make healthier choices. Additionally, yoga's stress-relieving properties help balance cortisol levels, a hormone linked to weight gain, especially around the midsection.

Furthermore, yoga poses target specific muscle groups, helping you tone and sculpt your body. As you flow through sequences like downward dog, plank, and warrior poses, you engage your core, arms, legs, and glutes, building strength and endurance. The balance and stability required in various poses also activate smaller stabilizer muscles, contributing to an overall toned physique.

To maximize weight loss and toning benefits, consider incorporating other forms of exercise into your routine. Pilates and core strengthening exercises complement yoga, focusing on building a strong core, enhancing posture, and improving flexibility. By combining these practices, you create a well-rounded fitness regimen that targets different muscle groups and promotes overall body strength.

In conclusion, yoga is a powerful tool for weight loss and toning that extends beyond physical benefits. Its mindful approach helps you develop a healthier relationship with your body and food, while the asanas and breathing techniques promote strength and flexibility. So, roll out your mat, breathe deeply, and embark on a transformative journey towards achieving a fit and balanced body through yoga.

Incorporating Strength Training in Your Yoga Routine

As adults, we often find ourselves juggling multiple responsibilities and struggling to maintain a healthy balance in our lives. Our bodies may feel stiff and weak, lacking the strength and flexibility we once had. That's where the combination of yoga and strength training can truly work wonders.

Yoga is renowned for its ability to improve flexibility, balance, and overall well-being. However, by incorporating strength training into your yoga routine, you can take your practice to the next level. Not only will you enhance your physical strength, but you'll also deepen your mind-body connection and cultivate mindfulness.

One effective way to incorporate strength training into your yoga routine is by using resistance bands or weights. These tools can be easily integrated into various yoga poses, allowing you to challenge your muscles and build strength. For instance, while in a warrior II pose, you can extend your arms out and hold a resistance band, engaging your upper body muscles and improving your arm strength.

Another great option is to practice yoga sequences that focus on strength-building poses. Poses such as chair pose, plank, and crow pose require a significant amount of strength to hold and maintain. By consciously engaging your muscles in these challenging positions, you not only build strength but also develop endurance and stability.

Incorporating Pilates and core-strengthening exercises into your yoga routine is yet another effective way to enhance your overall fitness. Pilates exercises, with their emphasis on core strength, can complement your yoga practice by targeting the deep muscles of your abdomen, back, and pelvis. This integration will not only improve your yoga performance but also enhance your posture, stability, and overall body awareness.

Mind-body connection and mindfulness are essential aspects of both yoga and flexibility training. By incorporating strength training into your yoga routine, you can further deepen this connection. As you challenge your body with resistance and build strength, you learn to listen to your body's cues and move mindfully. This heightened awareness can help you prevent injuries and optimize your overall workout experience.

In conclusion, incorporating strength training into your yoga routine is an excellent way to enhance your practice and overall fitness. By utilizing resistance bands or weights, focusing on strength-building poses, and integrating Pilates exercises, you can build strength, improve flexibility, and cultivate mindfulness. Embrace the balance of strength and flexibility, and watch your yoga practice flourish.

Yoga for Improved Posture and Alignment

In today's fast-paced world, where many of us spend long hours sitting at desks or hunched over electronic devices, maintaining good posture and alignment can be a challenge. However, the ancient practice of yoga offers a holistic solution to this common problem. By incorporating yoga into your fitness routine, you can not only improve your posture but also enhance your overall well-being.

Flex and Flow: Yoga and Flexibility Training for Adults

Yoga is a powerful tool for correcting poor posture and alignment because it focuses on the body as a whole. Through a series of asanas (poses) and conscious breathing, yoga helps to strengthen the muscles that support your spine and align your body in a natural, balanced way. By practicing yoga regularly, you can gradually retrain your body to sit and stand with proper alignment, alleviating the strain on your back, neck, and shoulders.

One of the key benefits of yoga for posture improvement is increased body awareness. As you move through different poses, you become more attuned to your body's alignment and the sensations it experiences. This heightened awareness allows you to make adjustments in real-time, ensuring that you maintain proper posture throughout your practice and in your daily life.

In addition to aligning the physical body, yoga also cultivates a mind-body connection that promotes mindfulness and self-care. By focusing on the breath and being fully present in each pose, you develop a deep sense of awareness and relaxation. This mind-body connection extends beyond your yoga mat, helping you to carry the principles of good posture and alignment into your everyday activities.

Furthermore, yoga can complement other forms of exercise such as Pilates and core strengthening. By adding yoga to your fitness routine, you can enhance your core stability, flexibility, and balance, which are essential for maintaining good posture. The integration of yoga and Pilates allows for a comprehensive approach to strengthening and aligning the body, resulting in improved overall fitness.

In conclusion, incorporating yoga into your fitness routine can greatly benefit your posture and alignment. By practicing yoga regularly, you can strengthen the muscles that support your spine, increase body awareness, and cultivate a mind-body connection. This holistic approach to posture improvement not only enhances your physical well-being but also contributes to your overall sense of mindfulness and self-care. So, roll out your yoga mat and embark on a journey of improved posture, alignment, and well-being.

Chapter 12: Integrating Yoga and Flexibility Training into Your Daily Life

Finding Balance in a Busy World

In today's fast-paced and demanding world, finding balance can seem like an elusive goal. As adults, we often find ourselves juggling multiple responsibilities, from work and family to personal commitments. The constant demands on our time and energy can leave us feeling overwhelmed and disconnected from ourselves. Fortunately, there is a solution – yoga and flexibility training.

Flex and Flow: Yoga and Flexibility Training for Adults

Yoga and flexibility training offer a holistic approach to finding balance in our lives. These practices not only help us develop physical strength and flexibility but also cultivate mental clarity and emotional well-being. By incorporating yoga and flexibility training into our daily routines, we can create a harmonious relationship between our bodies and minds, enabling us to navigate the challenges of a busy world with grace and ease.

One of the key benefits of yoga and flexibility training is their ability to improve physical strength and flexibility. Through a series of postures and stretches, these practices help to lengthen and strengthen our muscles, promoting better posture and alignment. As we become more flexible, we also reduce the risk of injury and improve our overall physical performance. Whether you're a beginner or an experienced practitioner, yoga and flexibility training offer a wide range of exercises and techniques to suit your individual needs and goals.

Beyond physical fitness, yoga and flexibility training also foster a deep mind-body connection. By focusing on our breath and being fully present in each moment, we learn to cultivate mindfulness and self-awareness. This heightened sense of awareness allows us to tune into our bodies' needs and listen to our intuition. As we become more in tune with ourselves, we can make conscious choices that support our overall well-being, both on and off the mat.

In a world that often glorifies busyness and productivity, finding balance can feel like an uphill battle. However, by incorporating yoga and flexibility training into our lives, we can reclaim our sense of balance and harmony. These practices offer a sanctuary amidst the chaos, allowing us to reconnect with ourselves and find peace in the present moment. So, take a moment to step onto your mat or engage in a flexibility training routine, and discover the transformative power of finding balance in a busy world.

Incorporating Yoga into Your Morning Routine

As adults, we often find ourselves rushing through our mornings, frantically trying to get ready for the day ahead. However, by incorporating yoga into your morning routine, you can start your day with a sense of calm and balance that will carry you through the rest of your day.

Yoga, known for its ability to improve flexibility, strength, and mindfulness, is the perfect practice to kickstart your morning. By dedicating just a few minutes each morning to yoga, you can reap the benefits throughout the day, both physically and mentally.

One of the main advantages of incorporating yoga into your morning routine is its ability to wake up your body and mind. The gentle stretching and flowing movements of yoga help to increase blood flow and oxygenation, leaving you feeling refreshed and energized. This can be especially beneficial for those who struggle with morning grogginess or stiffness.

In addition to the physical benefits, yoga also promotes a strong mind-body connection. By focusing on your breath and being present in the moment, you can cultivate a sense of mindfulness that carries throughout your day. This can help you stay centered and focused, even during stressful moments.

To incorporate yoga into your morning routine, start by setting aside a specific time and space for your practice. This could be a corner of your bedroom or a peaceful spot in your living room. Prepare your space with a yoga mat, blocks, and any other props that you may need.

Begin your practice with a few rounds of sun salutations to warm up your body and connect with your breath. From there, you can explore a variety of yoga poses and sequences that target your specific needs. If you're looking to improve flexibility, focus on poses that stretch your major muscle groups. If you want to build strength and stability, incorporate poses that engage your core and balance.

Remember to listen to your body and modify poses as needed. It's important to start slowly and gradually increase the duration and intensity of your practice. As you become more comfortable with your morning yoga routine, you may even consider adding meditation or mindfulness exercises to further enhance your mind-body connection.

By incorporating yoga into your morning routine, you can set a positive tone for the rest of your day. Not only will you experience physical benefits, such as increased flexibility and strength, but you'll also cultivate a sense of mindfulness and connection that will carry you through any challenges that come your way. So, why not start tomorrow morning with a few minutes of yoga? Your body and mind will thank you.

Yoga and Flexibility Training for Better Sleep

In today's fast-paced world, getting a good night's sleep can often seem like an elusive dream. Stress, anxiety, and the demands of our daily lives can easily disrupt our sleep patterns, leaving us feeling tired and sluggish. However, there is a powerful tool that can help us achieve the restful sleep we so desperately need - yoga and flexibility training.

Yoga, known for its gentle movements and focus on breath, has been practiced for centuries to promote physical and mental well-being. It is not only a fantastic way to improve flexibility, but also a powerful practice to calm the mind and reduce stress. By incorporating yoga into your daily routine, you can create a conducive environment for a peaceful night's sleep.

Flexibility training, which is often overlooked in traditional fitness routines, plays a crucial role in improving sleep quality. Tight muscles can lead to discomfort and restlessness, making it difficult to relax and fall asleep. By incorporating flexibility exercises into your fitness regimen, you can release tension in your muscles, promoting a sense of ease and relaxation that is essential for a restorative sleep.

When it comes to sleep, the mind-body connection is paramount. Yoga and flexibility training not only help to improve physical flexibility but also cultivate mindfulness and awareness. By practicing yoga poses and engaging in flexibility exercises, you become more attuned to your body and its needs. This heightened self-awareness can help you identify and address any issues that may be interfering with your sleep, such as poor posture or muscle tightness.

In "Flex and Flow: Yoga and Flexibility Training for Adults," we delve into the world of yoga and flexibility training, offering a comprehensive guide to improving sleep quality. Whether you are a yoga enthusiast or someone new to the practice, this book is designed to cater to adults seeking a holistic approach to fitness and well-being.

Within these pages, you will find a variety of yoga poses and flexibility exercises specifically curated to enhance sleep. From gentle stretching routines to targeted sequences that help alleviate stress and anxiety, you will discover a range of tools to support a peaceful night's rest.

If you are someone who is passionate about yoga and flexibility training, Pilates and core strengthening, or the mind-body connection and mindfulness in fitness, "Flex and Flow" is the ideal resource to deepen your understanding and enhance your practice. Join us on this transformative journey and unlock the secrets to a restful and rejuvenating sleep.

Conclusion: Embracing a Flexible and Mindful Lifestyle

In this journey through Flex and Flow: Yoga and Flexibility Training for Adults, we have explored the transformative power of embracing a flexible and mindful lifestyle. As adults seeking to enhance our well-being and achieve a higher level of fitness, we have delved into the realms of yoga and flexibility training, pilates and core strengthening, and the mind-body connection. Throughout this book, we have discovered the numerous benefits of incorporating these practices into our daily lives.

Flex and Flow: Yoga and Flexibility Training for Adults

Yoga and flexibility training have proven to be invaluable tools in improving our physical health, increasing our range of motion, and relieving muscle tension. By engaging in various yoga poses and flexibility exercises, we have learned to tune into our bodies, becoming more attuned to our body's needs and limitations. Through consistent practice, we have experienced increased flexibility, improved posture, and a greater sense of overall well-being.

Pilates and core strengthening have also played a significant role in our fitness journey. By focusing on strengthening the core muscles, we have developed a solid foundation for improved balance, stability, and overall body strength. The integration of pilates exercises into our fitness routine has not only helped us achieve a more toned physique but has also enhanced our performance in other physical activities.

However, it is essential to recognize that true well-being extends beyond physical fitness. The mind-body connection and mindfulness in fitness have emerged as crucial aspects of our journey. By cultivating a mindful approach to our workouts, we have learned to be present in the moment, fully engaging our minds and bodies. This heightened awareness has allowed us to connect with our inner selves, reduce stress, and find a sense of calm and tranquility amidst the chaos of everyday life.

Flex and Flow: Yoga and Flexibility Training for Adults

As we conclude this book, let us remember that embracing a flexible and mindful lifestyle is not a destination but an ongoing journey. It requires dedication, perseverance, and a willingness to explore new possibilities. By incorporating yoga, flexibility training, pilates, and mindfulness into our lives, we empower ourselves to live a life of balance and vitality.

So, dear readers, let us continue to foster a commitment to our physical and mental well-being. Let us embrace a flexible and mindful lifestyle with open hearts and open minds. May we continue to grow, evolve, and thrive on this transformative journey, bringing harmony and joy to every aspect of our lives.

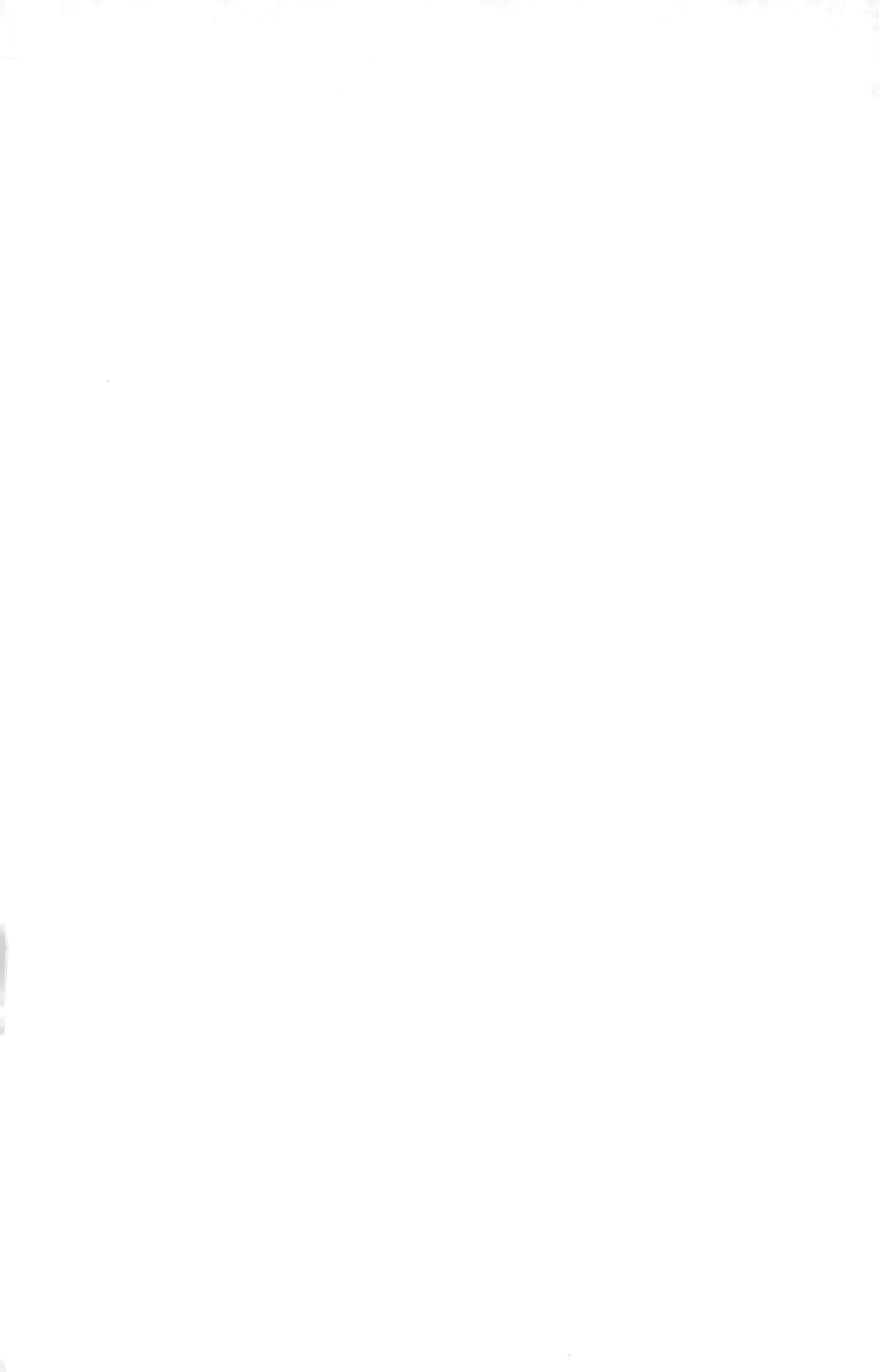